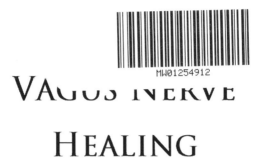

MW01254912

VAGUS NERVE

HEALING

Easy and Inexpensive Vagus Nerve
Stimulating Exercises That Activate
Your Body's Natural Self-Healing Power

PAUL COOGAN

Table of Contents

Introduction

The Vagus nerve has been getting a lot of attention lately as it has been used to treat conditions such as epilepsy, depression, anxiety, PTSD, and cluster headaches or chronic migraines. It is stimulated by a series of controlled electrical impulses delivered to the Vagus nerve. This is usually done medically where a device is inserted beneath a person's skin with a wire that connects it to the Vagus nerve.

A person's mental health has the ability to negatively affect and impact their physical health. People who have had chronic trauma often suffer from seizures, stomach and gastric upsets, autoimmune disorders, impulse control, and migraines. This is because everything is connected to the body's nervous system so when one part is not functioning correctly it can have a knock-on effect on another part of the body.

The nervous system is meant to flow in a rhythmic state which, in turn, allows the body to function normally, like getting enough sleep, having healthy digestion, being able to concentrate, being energetic, having a healthy immune system and a good state of mind, etc. Feeling tired, rundown, moody, constantly getting angry for no reason, living in fear, are all triggers that mean your system is out of rhythm, and this can affect all aspects of your health.

Not everyone can go and have a vagus nerve stimulator surgically implanted in their chest, nor should they have to. Your body is an amazing machine, and even though you may not feel like it is at the moment, with the correct exercises and stimulation to the vagus nerve, you may just be able to improve your health bit by bit.

Stimulating the vagus nerve can help the body learn to effectively cope and respond to various psychological and emotional stimuli. The good news is that you can stimulate the vagus nerve naturally with a few simple exercises every day or every other day. Stimulating the vagus nerve can be beneficial to a person's health.

In this book, you will be introduced to the nervous system to gain a basic understanding of the moving parts as well as how they fit together and work. A basic understanding of the nervous system will help you see the importance of the vagus nerve and how it can either positively or negatively affect your everyday wellbeing.

Through a series of exercises, that have been specially selected to be the most beneficial, you may just be able to stimulate your body's natural ability to heal, so you can start to solve your related health issues and improve your well-being for a better, healthier life.

Chapter 1:

THE HUMAN NERVOUS SYSTEM

To understand the importance of the vagus nerve and how it can affect your health, you first need to have a basic understanding of the human nervous system.

The Human Nervous System

The human nervous system has many working parts which are divided into two main sections:

- The central nervous system (CNS)

- The peripheral nervous system (PNS)

The nervous system is basically the body's main network operating system. The two main components of the network are the brain and the spinal cord which make up the central nervous system (CNS).

The Central Nervous System (CNS)

The Brain

The brain is the core part of the operating system. It controls our thoughts, stores our memories and emotions, mediates sensory perceptions, and controls both involuntary actions and voluntary actions. It is what drives our body and ensures all the systems in it work to keep the human body operational.

The brain is divided up into six sections:

- **The cerebrum**

The cerebrum is the largest part of the brain and runs from the temple through to the back of the skull, it is the top portion of the brain. The cerebrum has two sections, the left hemisphere and the right hemisphere. The cerebrum has four lobes:

- The **frontal lobe** — found at the front portion of the cerebrum — this is the lobe that manages and processes thought and reasoning.

- The **parietal lobe** — found in the middle of the cerebrum, positioned after the frontal lobe — this is the lobe that manages and processes sensory information.

- The **temporal lobe** — found below the frontal and parietal lobes, one either side of the cerebrum, near the region around the ears — this is the lobe that manages and processes hearing.

- The **occipital lobe** — found at the back of the cerebrum positioned after the parietal lobe — this is the lobe that manages and processes sight.

- **The cerebellum**

The cerebellum can be found just above the first cervical vertebrae of the neck, below the cerebrum and at the back of the skull. The cerebellum is what manages and processes:

- Balance

- Coordination

- Muscle tone

- Posture

- **The diencephalon**

This is the portion of the brain that is surrounded by the cerebrum, it sits above the midbrain. There are two sections to the diencephalon:

- The thalamus — responsible for transmitting sensory impulses to the cerebrum.

- The hypothalamus — controls the functions of the autonomic nervous system. It regulates and controls:

  - The dilation and constriction of blood vessels

  - Appetite

  - Water balance

  - Temperature

  - Sleep

  - Anger

  - Pain

  - Fear

  - Pleasure

- ■ Affection

- ● The midbrain

The midbrain is located on the top of the brain stem, it is responsible for the reflexes of the eye and ear.

- ● The pons

The pons is located in the brainstem just below the midbrain, it is responsible for reflex actions such as:

  - ○ Tasting

  - ○ The production of saliva

  - ○ Chewing

- ● The medulla oblongata

The medulla oblongata is found at the bottom of the brainstem, it is the section that connects the brain to the spinal cord. The medulla oblongata is responsible for regulating:

  - ○ Blood pressure

- ○ Blood vessel function

- ○ Coughing

- ○ Digestion

- ○ Heartbeat

- ○ Respiration

- ○ Sneezing

- ○ Swallowing

The Spinal Cord

The spinal cord is what connects the brain to the body. It is the pathway that passes information between the brain and the nerves found throughout the body.

It has 4 main sections to it:

- **Cervical** — this is the top half of the spinal cord which starts at the base of the skull and forms part of the neck.

- **Thoracic** — this is the part of the spinal cord that starts below the cervical section and forms the upper back, this is the section between the neck and the lower back.

- **Lumbar** — this is part of the lower back and is found below the thoracic section of the spinal cord.

- **Spinal nerves** — afferent and efferent spinal nerves — these are a series of nerves that extend from the spinal cord to the other parts of the body. These afferent and efferent nerves combine to make up the **peripheral nerves** which form the **peripheral nervous system.**

  ○ Afferent spinal nerves — these are the nerves that send information from the body to the brain.

  ○ Efferent spinal nerves — these are the nerves that send information from the brain to the rest of the body.

Neurons

Each and every region in the brain and spinal cord (CNS) is made up of many, many cells that are called neurons. Neurons transmit electrochemical signals in order to communicate with other parts of the body.

Normal cells and neurons do not look alike, although they are each made up of similar components. Neurons are made up of the following three parts:

- **Cell Body** — this is the core of the neuron and where the nucleus of the cell is housed. The nucleus is the control center of any cell.

- **Dendrites** — these structures look a bit like roots that extend out from the cell body. The dendrites are the structures that receive signals from the axons of other neurons.

- **Axon** - this is a structure that looks like a long tail, it is what conducts the electrical signals to other neurons, glands, and muscles in the body.

The human body contains around 86 billion neurons that form a complex network of communication channels from various parts of the body to the spinal cord and brain, as well as from the spinal cord and brain to the body. Up until the late 1990s, it was believed that neurogenesis - the process of forming new neurons - only occurred in humans from the time of conception up until the age of 3. After 3 years of age, it was through that neurogenesis stopped or slowed down. However, researchers at Princeton University found that neurogenesis did actually occur in certain parts of the adult brain.

Neurons do not all look alike, they can differ in structure, shape, and size depending on their use. But they are all made up of the same three parts.

There are three main types of neurons found in the nervous system:

- **Interneurons** — these are the most common types of neurons and can be found in the spinal cord and the brain. They are the neurons that pass information from one set of neurons in the spinal cord and brain on to another set of neurons if needed.

For example:

- ○ You get a paper cut - your sensory neurons send a signal to the interneuron.

- ○ The interneuron sends a signal to your motor neurons which is why you jerk your hand away.

- ○ The interneuron sends another signal to your brain and this is why you feel pain.

- **Motor neurons** — they are the neurons that communicate commands from the spinal cord and brain in order to let them send the signals to the necessary muscles and organs.

For example:

- ○ When you swallow, your motor neurons send a message to the interneurons that in

14

turn send the necessary signals from the brain and onto the muscles needed to enable you to swallow.

- **Sensory neurons** — these are the neurons responsible for communicating various sensations to the brain. Sensations such as:

  - Hearing

  - Sight

  - Smell

  - Taste

  - Touch

Glial Cells

The nervous system also contains cells that support the neurons and they are called glial cells. They do not actively process information and instead only support the neurons. There are just as many if not more glial cells in the brain than there are neurons.

There are five different types of glial cells:

- **Astrocyte** — star-shaped cells found in the CNS — get rid of brain debris or consume bits of dead neurons, carry nutrients to the neurons, and keep the neurons in position. They create a blood-brain barrier and have reparative functions.

- **Microglia** — found in the CNS — they aid the neuron by digesting parts of the neuron that has died off.

- **Oligodendroglia** — found in the CNS — they form tube-like structures called myelin sheaths that support and protect nerves in the central nervous system.

- **Satellite cells** —cells found in the PNS - these cells offer physical support to the neurons that are found in the peripheral nervous system.

- **Schwann cells** — cells found in the PNS — they are similar in both look and function to oligodendroglia cells but the Schwann cells (myelin) provide support to the nerves in the peripheral nervous system.

Peripheral Nervous System (PNS)

The central nervous system only consists of the brain and spinal cord. In order for the central nervous system to be able to regulate and control the functions of the rest of the body, it needs the help of the peripheral nervous system (PNS).

The central nervous system (CNS) relies on the peripheral nervous system (PNS) to capture and relay messages to organs, muscles, and glands. The messages are captured and either sent to the brain or from the brain to the rest of the body by the nerves.

The peripheral nervous system is divided into two main sections:

- The somatic nervous system

- The autonomic nervous system

The Somatic Nervous System

The main responsibility of the somatic nervous system is to relay information that pertains to sensory and motor functions of the body to and from the central nervous system. It sends these signals through the:

- Afferent sensory neurons that receive information from the nerves and relays the information to the central nervous system (brain and spinal cord).

- The efferent motor neurons collect information from the central nervous system and relay the information to muscle fibers throughout the body.

The somatic nervous system is made up of peripheral nerve fibers that start at either the brain or spinal cord and then extend to a muscle in the body, the skin, or a sensory organ.

The cell of the nerve fiber is usually located either in the brain or spinal cord. From there it extends to the skeletal muscles by means of a long thread-like structure called an axon. Where the axon meets the muscle fiber it synapses (connects) and forms a join or junction, when it joins with a muscle fiber the junction is called a neuromuscular junction.

The somatic nervous system is what controls voluntary movement, actions, and reflexes. They are the nerves that we can actively control so we can run, jump, swim, skip, hop, wave, dance, etc. It is the system that processes what we see, hear, touch, and smell.

The Autonomic Nervous System (ANS)

The autonomic nervous system is broken down into three sections:

- Sympathetic
    - This is the part of the nervous system that is responsible for the release of adrenaline that floods your veins when you encounter a "fight or flight" situation. It controls

stimuli such as excitement, anger, fear, stress, danger, etc.

○ It is a vital part of human survival, as it is the system that spurs the body into action when it is confronted with danger.

- **Parasympathetic**

    ○ This is the part of the nervous system that is responsible for the feelings of contentment when you are relaxing, eating, sleeping, and in a nice mellow state. It is known as the "rest and digest" reflex of the body.

    ○ It is also the system that helps the body stabilize and bring all the systems back into a calmer state after a "fight or flight" reflex.

- **Enteric Nervous system**

    ○ Often called the "brain in the gut" or "the second brain" because it works independently of the CNS while still staying connected to the CNS by communicating through the autonomic nervous system.

- o It is the gastrointestinal system's own nervous system.

- o The enteric nervous system communicates to both the brain and the immune system. But it can work efficiently independently from them.

- o Studies have shown that the enteric nervous system continues to function even if the Vagus nerve is severed.

- o The enteric nervous system holds 5 times more neurons than the spinal cord.

Although there are three sections to the autonomic nervous system, the enteric nervous system is usually not grouped with the sympathetic and parasympathetic nervous system. Not much is known about the enteric nervous system but research scientists at Duke University found a way to start getting a closer look at the system in 2016.

If we take the polyvagal theory into account, we would further breakdown the autonomic nervous system into another section called the 'Social engagement system'. The social engagement system would then be the system on which the sympathetic or parasympathetic nervous systems would base their response triggers.

Chapter 2:

THE POLYVAGAL THEORY

The Polyvagal Theory was proposed by Dr. Stephen Proges in 1994, where he theorized that there are links between social behavior and the autonomic nervous system. Over the years, the theory has gained ground and a lot of attention with new treatments being developed each day linked to treating various mental and physical disorders associated with vagus nerve stimulation.

How the Brain Responds to Stressful Situations

The autonomic nervous system is the system that keeps humans alive by controlling what we think of as our basic instincts. If you touch a hot plate on the stove, you are going to instantly pull your hand away. That is your autonomic nervous system responding to danger. If someone physically threatens you, your first instinct is to either flee or fight which is the body's basic survival instinct.

The Stress Alarm

When a stressful situation is encountered, the sensory organs such as the eyes, ears, or both send a signal to the amygdala. The amygdala is found near the hippocampus in the frontal lobe of the brain. Its name is actually Greek for almond as it is an almond-shaped structure that is responsible for the processing of emotion. Each human has two amygdalae, one in each hemisphere of the cerebrum.

The amygdala can be likened to a lookout tower such as that of a forest fire station that ensures everything that may be the start of a forest fire is reported so it can be further investigated.

The amygdala processes the information it has been sent by the eyes and ears, these will be images and sounds. If it perceives any of this information as a threat it will send alarm signals to the hypothalamus.

The hypothalamus, which is found in the diencephalon part of the brain, in turn, triggers the sympathetic nervous system to respond to the threat. This signal gets sent through the autonomic nervous system and activates the adrenal glands that release adrenaline (epinephrine) into the body through the bloodstream.

The release of adrenaline into the bloodstream causes the heartbeat to increase. This, in turn, pumps blood to the heart, vital organs, and muscles a lot faster increasing blood pressure and a person's pulse. When adrenaline is pumping through the body, a person will experience rapid breathing as the small airways in the lungs are forced wide open. The increase in oxygen to the brain makes it more alert as well as sharpening your instincts, vision, and hearing. As these functions are becoming enhanced, the adrenaline is also creating more energy for the body by using stored fats and glucose to release fuel into the bloodstream.

This may sound like a long process in theory but in practice, it all happens in a split second and usually before the conscious mind has time to process the threat. That is why you will jump out of the way of imminent danger, as soon as you feel the heat you will pull away, etc.

Winding down After the Threat Has Passed

After the threat has passed, you feel like you are zinging, your hands are probably shaking, you may even feel a bit giddy, as your heart pounds. Then slowly your body will start to relax as the parasympathetic system of the autonomic nervous system takes over. Because it has received signals from the hypothalamus that the threat has passed, the parasympathetic system releases a hormone called acetylcholine.

This is the hormone that slows the heart rate down in order to bring the body back to a normal rhythm and balance out the stress level. This is called maintaining homeostasis.

Homeostasis

Homeostasis in the human body refers to the body's ability to maintain a modicum of internal and external balance when faced with various environmental challenges or changes.

As humans have evolved, one of the main systems that has remained the same is the body's survival instinct. As times have changed, this instinct has had to adapt to different types of environmental challenges and changes. Being able to successfully maintain a state of homeostasis when faced with adversity is very important to maintaining physical and mental health as well as overall survival.

This does not only mean being able to successfully defend oneself physically, it also means the body's internal abilities to cope with stress. Its ability to release certain hormones when it should, to be able to switch from one state (mobilize for flight or flight) to the other (relax and digest) successfully.

How the Human Body Maintains Homeostasis

- When you are hot you sweat — this is the body's way of cooling itself down.

- When you are cold you shiver — this is the body's way of trying to get warm.

- When you are feeling tired or groggy you yawn — the brain needs oxygen to stay alert, yawing draws in more oxygen to feed the brain.

- If there is too much glucose in the system, the body releases insulin — the body needs to maintain optimum levels of glucose in order to keep healthy and ensure certain organs do not get damaged.

- If there is a bacterial infection the lymphatic system spurs into action — the lymphatic system fights off the bacteria to stop a person from getting sick.

- If blood pressure is too high, the body releases hormones to slow down the heart rate — high blood pressure is usually a result of high heart rate.

- If blood pressure is too low, the body will increase the heart rate — low blood pressure is usually due to a low heart rate.

- Maintaining proper oxygen levels in the system through breathing is monitored and managed by the nervous system.

- The urinary and digestive tract are ways that the body can get rid of ingested toxins by urinating or defecating.

What Is the Polyvagal Theory?

To understand the polyvagal theory, you must first understand the sympathetic and parasympathetic systems of the autonomic nervous system.

Sympathetic Nervous System vs Parasympathetic Nervous System

The sympathetic nervous system is the system that mobilizes the body into action in response to a threat. A threat could be anything from getting a bad feeling about someone you have just met, being anxious about work or having to get on a flight, fear, stress, etc.

The parasympathetic nervous system is the system that stabilizes the body after it has had a stimulating response to a situation, in other words, it is the brakes that slow the sympathetic response down. For instance, it is a system that helps to slow down the heart rate after you have gone for a run or any other form of activity during which you've exerted yourself. It helps the body calm down after receiving a shock or coming under threat of an attack, or after you have been put under high stress. It is what calms you down after an angry episode.

The parasympathetic nervous system is mostly controlled and regulated by the most predominant nerve in the body's nervous system, the vagus nerve.

The Polyvagal Theory

According to the polyvagal theory, the sympathetic and parasympathetic systems of the autonomic nervous system respond differently to various signals depending on whether the body is under stress (feeling unsafe) or functioning normally (feeling safe). These signals are given off from another system of the autonomic nervous system called the 'social engagement system'.

The polyvagal theory is based on how the body handles stress in accordance with the ever-changing environment around it and its ability to maintain homeostasis.

Through a process called 'neuroperception', the social engagement system is constantly scanning the environment to determine whether there is a threat or not.

A Breakdown of How the System Works Under Stressful Conditions

1. At the social engagement level:

   a. The neuroperception scans the environment for changes and then determines whether those changes pose a threat or not.

   b. The social engagement system is responsible for a person's facial expressions, voice, heartbeat, and breathing.

   c. What the body may perceive as a threat is dependent on the person, as what some might fear, others might not.

d. Snakes are a good example to use to explain this theory. Since people who know about snakes will know which ones pose a threat and which don't, they would know that a slug eater will be harmless to them and therefore not a threat. But others who do not know about snakes will see a slug eater as a snake, and snakes mean danger, therefore they are a threat.

2. If the social engagement system perceives a threat, before it alerts any other systems, it will try to resolve the threat by means of **communication or reasoning**.

   Here it is normal for the person to:

   - Try appeasement

   - Negotiate

   - Lie

   - Cheat

- Manipulate

- Become passive-aggressive

- Try to ignore or deny the situation

3. If communication or reasoning fails to calm the situation down so the body feels normal and safe, the social engagement system will signal the sympathetic system to take over.

4. **When the sympathetic system is triggered:**

   a. The first instinct it initiates is flight - leave the source of danger. For instance, putting your hand on a hot plate, you pull away from the danger. If the snake is not too close you will turn tail and run.

   b. If you cannot leave or get away from the source of danger or stress, the sympathetic system then triggers the fight response.

c. It triggers this response in order to protect the body from harm and allow it to defend itself.

d. The fight response is the **mobilization response** of the sympathetic system and it controls the movements of the arms, legs, and torso.

e. This is where you will see some people run toward the danger in order to get rid of it, or if someone takes a swing at you, you either duck or block and counteract.

5. If neither fight nor flight is an option, the sympathetic system signals the parasympathetic system and signals the situation as a life threat.

6. **As soon as the parasympathetic system is activated:**

a. In response to a life threat, it goes into **immobilization mode** which is the freeze response. It can also mean shock, fainting, and dissociation.

b. Like if a snake twined itself around your leg, your body detects the snake as life-threatening and you instantly freeze. You want to move but your body seems like it is paralyzed in place.

c. In an accident, your body will shut down in shock or you could pass out from it.

d. The **immobilization mode** is the body's way of protecting the person from pain in the face of death or to bring the body back to a normal state. For instance, when a person faints it gets the blood flowing again, the shock is the body's way of responding to traumatic situations.

7. The body will stay in a state of **mobilization** or **immobilization** until the threat dissipates and it feels safe or normal again.

A Breakdown of How the System Works Under Normal Conditions

1. **At the social engagement level**

   a. The neuroperception scans the environment for changes and then determines whether those changes pose a threat or not.

   b. In normal conditions a person would have a smile on their face, have a softer normal pitch to their voice, their heart rate would be normal as would their breathing.

   c. They would be relaxed and enjoying themselves.

2. **Even when in a normal state, the sympathetic system kicks in**

   a. Feeling comfortable, safe and in a normal state, a person can function at an everyday level and will be willing to socially engage or participate in activities such as:

- Work

- Singing

- Dancing

- Doing their favorite hobbies

- Sports

- Being intimate

- Socializing

b. Participation in such activities is the **mobilization state** of the normal sympathetic system function.

3. **The parasympathetic system is activated in the normal state** in response to our body's needed to relax and regenerate after a day of normal activities.

a. The parasympathetic system **immobilization mode** in the normal state ensures the body has:

- Rest

- Relaxation

- Regeneration

Shifting Environments Effects on the Nervous System from One State to the Other

Even when the body is at a peaceful, resting state, a shift in the environment can make it shift from one state to the other, for example:

- A body at sleep can awaken to a life-threatening situation.

  - The system goes from parasympathetic immobile rest to parasympathetic life threat mode. For example, you could wake up to someone trying to cause you harm.

  - The system can go from parasympathetic immobile rest to sympathetic fight or flight mode. For example, you could wake up to an unfamiliar noise.

- The system can go from parasympathetic immobile rest to sympathetic normal mobilization. In other words, you wake up in the morning and have to go to work.

Each state is capable of switching to the other as soon as the environment around you changes.

Chapter 3:

THE VAGUS NERVE

Now that you have a basic understanding of the nervous system and the polyvagal theory, you will be able to better understand the functions and importance of the vagus nerve.

The word "vagus" is Latin and means "wandering" which is an apt name for this nerve that wanders through the body starting at the brain, then through the neck organs, down in the chest, and into the stomach.

What is the Vagus Nerve?

The vagus nerve is the longest of the 12 cranial nerves in the human body, and it is one of the most complex nerves. It is also known as cranial nerve X (10). The Vagus nerve forms part of the autonomic nervous system which, in turn, forms part of the peripheral nervous system. The autonomic nervous system is what enables us to automatically do things like breathe, regulate blood pressure, etc. These are called involuntary actions.

Without the autonomic nervous system (ANS), we would have to consciously think about breathing all the time, think about keeping our heart beating and make our own blood vessels open and close. The ANS is also part of the nervous system that controls some involuntary reflex actions such as sneezing, vomiting, coughing, and swallowing.

The vagus nerve is part of the parasympathetic division of the autonomic nervous system. The vagus nerve makes up 75% of all the nerve fibers in the parasympathetic division of the autonomic nervous system. It is what connects the brainstem to the rest of the body so the brain can effectively monitor and communicate with cells, organs, muscles, etc. It is also the only nerve of this system that starts in the brainstem (medulla oblongata).

The vagus nerve is one of, if not the most, important nerves in the body as it contributes sensory and motor nerve fibers to the neck and everything from there down to the middle of the large intestine. This means the nerve has many responsibilities which we will discuss below.

What Are the Functions of the Vagus Nerve?

Responsibilities of the Vagus Nerve

- It transmits information about touch, temperature, and pain from the meninges near the back of the head to the outer and inner.

- It has a small role to play in tasting by transmitting the taste sensation from the root of the tongue and the epiglottis.

- Sensory information sent from the internal organs found in the chest, stomach, and neck is received by the vagus nerve. These are organs such as the heart, the digestive tract, and the esophagus.

- It also transmits information about any changes in blood pressure and the receptors that monitor changes in the oxygen levels in the blood.

- The vagus nerve plays an important role in how we swallow and speak by controlling the muscles of the soft palate, larynx, tongue muscle, and pharynx.

- It supplies nerves to organs in the abdomen, thorax, and neck. Thus, it has control over functions such as the slowing down of the heart after a person has received a fright, coughing, decreasing inflammation, lowering blood pressure, managing fear, and sending signals from the gut to the brain.

Dissecting the Vagus Nerve

The Vagus nerve starts in the medulla oblongata and not only feeds information to the brain but also carries information from the brain. The vagus nerve has two stems, one that appears from the left side of the medulla and the other from the right side. They are long thread-like fibers that are made up of a lot of smaller cells that send information from the brain to the rest of the body. They also receive information from the parts of the body they supply to send it through to the brain to process.

Although it is actually two nerves, the vagus nerve is only ever referred to as one nerve.

The information the vagus nerve carries into and out of the brain is fed by the different nuclei associated with the vagus nerve that can be found in the medulla. The type of nuclei is dependent on the information that is being transmitted by the vagus nerve:

- **The spinal trigeminal nucleus** — this nucleus carries information about pain, touch, and temperature.

- **The solitary nucleus** — this is where sensory information from the internal organs travels to.

- **The dorsal vagal motor nucleus** — this is where parasympathetic fibers originate from.

- **The nucleus ambiguous** — this is where parasympathetic fibers begin that extend to the heart. It is also where the motor signals for the vagus nerve originate from.

Damage to the Vagus Nerve

As the vagus nerve is the longest cranial nerve, there are a lot of places that can get damaged.

How the Vagus Nerve is Checked for Damage

It is best to get a medical professional to test for vagus nerve damage.

The way the check is to see if the person has a proper gag reflex. They will take a soft cotton swab and ask the patient to open wide in order to tickle both sides at the back of the throat. As everyone should know by now, if something tickles the uvula or the part of the throat near it, you should have an instant gag reflex. If there is little to no gag reflex, the doctor may order more tests as this could be a sign of vagal nerve damage.

Signs and Symptoms of Vagus Nerve Damage

As the vagus nerve is a very long nerve and supports a lot of organs, there can be many different indications of damage in different areas along the nerves.

Some of the symptoms that may indicate damage to the Vagus nerve can include:

- Hoarse voice

- Loss of voice completely

- Wheezing

- No gag reflex

- Trouble swallowing

- Earache

- Stomach acid abnormalities

- Bloating of the stomach

- Pain in the stomach

- Blood pressure problems

- Erratic heartbeat

- Vomiting

- Nausea

Conditions That May Be Caused by Vagus Nerve Damage

- **Gastroparesis**

Damage to the vagus nerve can affect the digestive system. It can cause the involuntary contractions to be less effective which stops the stomach from being able to be sufficiently empty out. This causes a backup in the digestive system and can make a person really ill; it can cause:

- Painful bloating of the abdomen as undigested food cause gaseous build-up

- Nausea and bad indigestion

- Vomiting - a person may bring up undigested food

- Weight loss

- Blood sugar fluctuations

- Loss of appetite

○ Always feeling full

- **Vasovagal syncope**

The vagus nerve stimulates the nerves which help the system to normalize itself after stimulation, such as slowing down the heart rate, dropping blood pressure, etc. Sometimes the vagus nerve will overreact to certain stimuli which can cause dizziness, passing out, or fainting.

A person will pass out when blood flow to the brain is restricted, and when this happens, the body loses consciousness. The body goes limp because it will also lose control over the muscles.

When the person falls over the blood flow is once again restored to the brain, which in turn returns the person to a state of consciousness.

What part does the vagus nerve play in passing out? It is the nerve that regulates both blood pressure by dropping it and the heart rate by slowing it down.

When the nerve overreacts to various stimuli it can make the blood pressure or heart rate drop too low.

Stimuli that can cause the vagus nerve to overreact and cause syncope:

- Certain visual stimulation like seeing blood

- Being out in the extreme heat

- Standing for long periods of time

- Fear

Treatment of a Damaged Vagus Nerve

Medical Treatments

Depending on what the damage is, they may need to treat it with various medications, or if the damage has caused Gastroparesis then the doctor may have you undergo pyloroplasty. This is a procedure that will relax and widen the pyloric valve which will allow the stomach to operate properly.

Natural Treatments

Sometimes the vagus nerve can be treated through natural methods that you can practice at home. In order to get the vagus nerve working again, you will need to stimulate it. Here are a few ways in which to stimulate the Vagus nerve, for a more in-depth solution, see **Chapter 5 - How to Naturally Stimulate the Vagus Nerve.**

- Breathing exercises

- Cold shower

- Massage

- Various physical exercises such a gym, running, walking, stretching, Tai chi, etc. can stimulate the nerve

- Acupuncture

Chapter 4:

VAGAL TONE

There has been a lot of research into the vagus nerve and its connection to a person's mental as well as physical health. Research shows that a vagus nerve that exhibits a high vagal tone has a positive impact on a person's mood as well as their physical well-being.

A well-toned vagus nerve will quickly return the body back to its normal or relaxed state after it has had a stressful encounter. This happens because the vagal nerve quickly reduces the heart rate, blood pressure, stress levels, has a positive impact on the brain and encourages healthy digestion when it slows to its relaxed state.

Research has even found that if a pregnant mother has a low vagal tone when her child is born, the child too will have a low vagal tone. The infant may also have lower levels of serotonin and dopamine than normal.

The Vagal Tone Index of the Vagus Nerve

Just like anything in the body the vagus nerve can get damaged, it can also overreact, and it can send faulty signals to the brain, i.e., it becomes dysfunctional.

The vagus nerve not only takes messages from the brain to the internal organs but also delivers messages from the internal organs to the brain. This means not only does the brain have control over the vagus nerve, but the nerve, in turn, can have an effect on brain function.

For example, there may be a bacterial infection in an organ regulated by the vagus nerve. The nerves in the organ send a message which is carried by the vagus nerve to the brain which causes it to affect a person's mood — you may feel horrible, sleepy, and just plain miserable.

As it is a long nerve that touches many parts of the body, there are many places that something can go wrong and cause a dysfunction of the vagus nerve. These places can be categorized according to the three main functions of the vagus nerve that can be susceptible to dysfunction.

Three Main Functions of the Vagus Nerve Susceptible to Dysfunction

- Direct communication to the brain.

- Delivering information from the brain to organs in the body.

- Delivering information for the organs in the body to the brain.

Signs and Symptoms of Vagus Nerve Dysfunction

- **Aggressive behavior**

There is nothing wrong with a bit of healthy aggression now and then. Especially when a person is being attacked. The problem is when there is a constant display of aggression.

Usually, when aggressive behavior is triggered the body is able to calm itself down. If there is a dysfunction in the vagal nerve however, the body constantly thinks it is under threat and so it keeps the body in its fight or flight mode.

- **Anxiety**

Everyone experiences a bit of anxiety, in this fast-paced world it is hard not to have some form of stress or pressure pushing down on you. A healthy vagus nerve has the ability to counteract the fight or flight mode caused by stress and calm the body back down to a normal state.

If a person is in a constant state of anxiety, the sympathetic nervous system keeps triggering hormones to help the body defend itself. However, the body can only tolerate a certain amount of these hormones before it starts to be severely affected by them. Just like you would be if you took too much of any substance.

- **Depression**

Depression is a hard disorder to control and manage as it causes a person to be in a constant state of feeling down, blue, sad, and to lose interest in just about everything. It can cause a person to behave erratically, have bad mood swings, and even contemplate or attempt suicide.

There are various processes in the brain that influence depressive disorders, and the vagus nerve is one of the influencers. But just as it can influence depression, studies have shown it can also help to alleviate depression.

- **Emotional**

When the vagus nerve is not working properly it affects your emotions. One minute you will feel fine, but the next you will feel all teary or you may get angry. If the body is stuck in the fight or flight mode it will keep releasing hormones, eventually, it is going to take a toll on your system. It can present as a person being over-emotional.

- **Painful inflamed joints**

The vagus nerve is part of the system that prevents inflammation by alerting the brain to the substances that cause inflammation. This then lets the brain send signals to the system that is responsible for fighting off the inflammation. If the vagus nerve is not functioning correctly, it cannot get this signal to the brain to fight proinflammatory cytokines so it cannot stop the inflammation reflex.

- **Constantly feeling dizzy**

If the vagus nerve is overstimulated it can drop the blood pressure or heart rate too low which can cause a person to feel dizzy and even in some cases faint. The vagus nerve is responsible for the constriction of blood vessels in order to slow down the heart rate and lower blood pressure after a stressful situation for the body.

- **Tired all the time**

When any part of your body is not functioning well it takes a toll on your system. A person feeling tired when their body is sick or when something has gone wrong is the body's defense mechanism to help fight off illness or to try and right itself. As it does this best when a person is asleep, you will feel tired and miserable.

- **Erratic heartbeat**

As the vagus nerve controls the heart rate, one that is not working correctly could make your heartbeat increase and then drop suddenly. This makes motions like walking, standing, and even sitting up difficult to do.

- **Irritable bowel syndrome, GERD, and indigestion**

The vagus nerve is the nerve that sends a signal to tell the brain that the gut needs to get ready to digest food when a person starts to chew. The food we are chewing starts to get broken down and as we swallow various acids break it down even more so that it is easy to digest. A faulty vagus nerve can cause this movement to slow down so that food takes longer to digest. This means acid build-up, waste products, and partially digested food start to cause all sorts of complications for the system. These complications can manifest as irritable bowel syndrome, gastroesophageal reflux disease (GERD), heartburn, and acid indigestion.

- **Passing out for no reason**

When the vagus nerve is overstimulated, it constricts the blood vessels, cutting off blood flow to the brain.

This causes a drop in heart rate and blood pressure which causes a person to pass out.

A dysfunctional vagus nerve may lead to a more serious condition if it is not treated. If you are exhibiting any of the signs above, you should seek advice from your doctor as if left untreated the issues can and probably will escalate.

Conditions That Could Arise from a Dysfunctional Vagus Nerve

- Dissociation

- Eating disorders

- Obsessive-compulsive disorder (OCD)

- Tinnitus

- Circulation problems

- Cluster and chronic migraine headaches

- Cancer

- Heart disease and chronic heart failure

- Leaky Gut Syndrome (LGS)

- Obesity

- Chronic mood swings

- Fibromyalgia

- A disorder that affects the memory such as Alzheimer's

The dysfunction of the vagal nerve or even damage to it is usually associated with lifestyle choices, disease, or physical damage to the nerve itself.

Diseases and Lifestyle Choices That Can Cause Dysfunction or Damage the Vagus Nerve

- **Diabetes**

Diabetes causes fluctuations in blood glucose levels which can damage the vagus nerve. This can lead to gastric problems as the vagus nerve controls how quickly the stomach gets emptied and diabetic damage to the nerve can cause gastroparesis. Gastroparesis is when the stomach does not empty completely.

- **Chronic fatigue syndrome and Fibromyalgia**

If the vagus nerve is dysfunctional or becomes damaged, it may misinterpret signals which can cause it to keep sending signals to the brain to shut down by sending out hormones that cause fatigue and pain.

- **Poor posture**

This can lead to constriction of the vagus nerve, which in turn, can lead to all sorts of physical problems such as poor digestion. This can lead to other internal problems for the system. Poor posture also leads to poor breathing and not getting enough oxygen into the blood can affect the vagus tone index.

- **Chronic stress and anxiety**

Chronic stress constantly puts pressure on the parasympathetic and sympathetic systems. The system will be in a constant state of switching on mobilization mode and then trying to switch off mobilization mode to bring the body back to normal. A state of constant stress is like flicking a light bulb on and off all the time, eventually, the bulb is going to blow. This is the same for people who are anxious all the time and live with constant worries that they cannot shut off.

- **Smoking**

Smoking causes a lot of problems for the nervous system. It damages the vagus nerve and the way it responds to cardiac signals, it also affects the lungs and other organs that the vagus nerve is responsible for.

- **Excessive intake of alcohol**

When the body consumes alcohol, it inhibits certain receptors in the brain, which causes vagal neuropathy. It reduces cardiac vagal tone which if continued to be abused will start to have serious effects on the rest of the nerve. As the nerve touches many organs in the body it could have a knock-on effect.

- **Physical damage to any part of the vagus nerve**

If parts of the vagus nerve get damaged it can cause serious mental and physical issues. The nerve can be damaged through injury or by various diseases. Seizures have been known to cause damage to the vagus nerve

In order to help the nerve recover or keep it healthy, a person needs to consider their lifestyle and commit to making some changes in order to improve their quality of life by increasing their vagal tone index. Vagal tone represents the activity of the vagus nerve, the better the tone, the faster the body reverts back to a normal or relaxed state from a stressful situation.

Implement a Few Lifestyle Changes to Start Increasing Vagal Nerve Health

- **Cut down on alcohol consumption**

Alcohol affects the Vagus nerve by spiking it into activity. This can cause erratic heartbeats, and if too much alcohol is consumed, it can and will end up damaging the nerve. A glass of wine at night may be fine, it could even have a positive effect on your heart. However, overdoing it leads to all sorts of problems, a lot of them may stem from the damage caused to the vagus nerve for alcoholism.

- **Get more exercise**

Exercise is essential for all parts of the body, not just the vagus nerve. But it is a great way to increase vagal tone and ensure the vagus nerve is functioning at its best. Dunking your face in cold water after strenuous exercises that have raised the body's temperature sets the vagus nerve in action.

- **Get more sleep**

It might seem that the answer to a lot of health problems is to get more sleep and there is a reason for that. Sleep is the time that your body gets to sort out problems, reset, and fight off nasty intruders into the system looking to do it harm. That is why, when there is a problem in the body, the vagus nerve will send signals to the brain to produce the hormones that make a person sleepy. While the body is at rest it is usually calm with minimal threat to it. This is the time when all the administration on the body begins. Kind of like what happens when a place shuts down for maintenance or how buildings are cleaned at night when no one is around. The next morning, you get to your office and it is all sparkling clean and ready for you to use.

The body has many working parts, which means it has a lot to do, including making sense of and storing away information you have taken in during the day. So, it needs a good 8 hours to get this done. Interruptions in the sleep pattern interrupt the body's functions. Soon, these escalate into bigger and bigger physical as well as mental issues.

It is also not just about getting enough sleep it is about getting enough quality sleep. This means making sure your sleeping environment is conducive to getting a good night's rest. In **Chapter 5,** there is a section on how to make your sleeping environment sleep worthy.

Take note of how you sleep as well because sleep posture (yes, that is a thing), is really important to getting quality sleep, it also has an impact on the rest that your body receives.

- **Eat more fiber**

Eating more fiber is not just for people of advanced age who need digestive aid. It is for everyone. Fiber has been known to increase a hormone called GLP-1, and this hormone helps to slow down the emptying of the stomach to help you feel fuller longer. It is also a hormone that is important for helping communication between the vagus nerve and the brain.

This does not mean that you must go and eat copious amounts of fiber. It simply means that you should make sure you have at least the recommended daily amount that suits your body's needs.

- **Add more seafood to your diet**

Fish has always been said to be brain food, and that is because it is. A research study was done in 2014 that appeared in the American Journal of Preventive Medicine. The scientists found that fish increased grey matter in the brain. Particularly in the areas where Alzheimer's first tends to appear.

Eicosapentaenoic acid (EPA) and docosahexaenoic acid (DHA), both types of omega-3 fatty acids, are found in fish and help to stimulate the Vagus nerve and increase vagal tone. If you do not like fish, you can use fish oil supplements.

- **Have intermittent bouts of fasting**

The vagus nerve is a very busy nerve that is communicating with various parts of the body every single day, 24/7, 365 days a year. It is the go-between for communication between these parts and the central nervous system. One of its main functions is to regulate the digestive system. Fasting every now and then helps with a lot of things in the body like metabolism and regulating weight control. It also gives the vagus nerve a little rest so it can pay more attention to its other responsibilities. Intermittent fasting can also improve vagal tone.

- **Sunlight exposure or Vitamin D supplements**

Get more sunlight by spending time outside and soaking up the sun. Not too much sun though. What the sun does is gives us vitamin D, and vitamin D is very important for cardiovascular autonomic nerve function. As the vagus nerve is responsible for ensuring the heart rhythm is correct, vitamin D is essential for it to operate correctly.

- **Meditate**

Try and incorporate meditation into your day at least 2 to 3 times a week. Meditation has been known to slow down the heart rate and decrease blood pressure as it relieves stress and anxiety.

- Have a cold shower or splash your face with cold water often

Take a cold shower every now and then and splash cold water on your face at least once or twice a day. This stimulates most of the nerves and shocks the body into a response that stimulates the vagus nerve.

- Get a massage on a regular basis

Anything from a foot massage to a full body massage is good for stimulating the vagus nerve and getting the blood flowing to areas of your skin and body.

- Add zinc to your diet

Most people do not even realize they are zinc deficient, and it is crucial to the function of the vagus nerve. Try to supplement your diet with the recommended daily dose of zinc.

- Add serotonin to your diet

Serotonin has been known to activate various receptors that activate the vagus nerve. Speak to a pharmacist or medical professional about how to increase your serotonin and implement their suggestions into your lifestyle.

- **Have probiotics on a regular basis**

Gut health is important for the vagus nerve and keeping it healthy is a good way to increase vagal tone. Find a good probiotic by speaking to your pharmacist or medical advisor.

- **Try pulsed electromagnetic field therapy**

Although there are devices you can use by yourself at home, you do not want to overstimulate your vagus nerve. So, the use of these devices should be done under the strict supervision of your medical advisor. There have been some good outcomes with the use of these devices.

- **Get out more and socialize**

Believe it or not, socializing is a great way to increase vagal tone and get the vagus nerve stimulated. There are all sorts of benefits to mental health from socializing as humans are, by nature, social creatures. So, it stands to reason that limiting yourself or cutting off social contact altogether will be detrimental to our health.

Socializing helps build up our 'social-behavioral system' by fine-tuning it and making it more robust. Kind of like exercising your muscles builds up muscle tone, socializing helps build up a natural coping mechanism and thickens our hides so to speak.

- **Smile and laugh often**

If you are going to socialize more, then you should definitely make sure you smile and laugh more. There is a ton of research easily accessible to everyone about the health benefits of a smile and a full belly laugh. It not only has health benefits for the body, mind, and soul, it is also good for your social health. A person with a smile on their face is a lot more approachable and attractive.

Laughing and smiling are also a great way to increase vagal tone as they positively stimulate the vagus nerve.

- **Dance and sing whenever you can**

Dancing is a great feel-good way to stimulate the vagus nerve and music is a good way to get the energy flowing. Singing and humming vibrate and stimulate the vagus nerve into action. It is a good way to exercise the back of the throat and increase vagal tone. So, sing loud and strong as you dance like no one is watching you.

- **Acupuncture**

Try acupuncture as it is a great way to both stimulate and strengthen the vagus nerve. See **Chapter 5** for a bit more information on how acupuncture can help with the vagus nerve.

It is important to know that acupuncture can also overstimulate the vagus nerve, so it is very important to vet the acupuncturist well. Make sure they are experienced and have performed the procedure many times. It is also important to consult with your medical professional before trying it, especially if you have a preexisting condition.

Vagal Tone Measurement

A high heart rate variability usually means your vagal tone will be high too, this is measured by your heart rate and your breathing rate. The vagal tone can be increased by either having a medical device surgically inserted beneath your skin that sends electrical impulses to the vagus nerve or you can work on toning it naturally.

There is a device that can help you monitor and manage your heart rate variability (HRV) called the EmWave2. This device is also used by medical or scientific professionals in order to monitor and measure the vagal tone for both consulting and research purposes. If you are going to use any devices that monitor or have anything to do with the heart or blood pressure you should always seek advice from a trained, qualified medical professional first.

Stimulating the vagus nerve has been shown to be helpful in treating a few mental health issues and brain disorders.

Vagus Nerve Stimulation for Mental Health and Brain Conditions

- **Anxiety**

Anxiety is the feeling of having constant worries that escalate to a point where the person no longer feels in control of them. This leads to sheer panic and could bring about panic disorder.

People get anxious due to many different things, such as paying bills on time, worrying about their kids traveling on the school bus, having to get on a flight, and so on.

When a person is anxious, the body goes into its mobilization mode and triggers the fight or flight response. This releases various hormones into the system, and while a person is still anxious, the body continues to try and defend itself, so the parasympathetic system does not get a chance to bring the body back to a normal state.

With so many fight or flight hormones coursing through a person's veins, the mind is in a constant state of danger awareness so small things can seem like mountains. This can and usually does at some point lead to a full-blown panic attack.

The stimulation of the vagus nerve can trigger the parasympathetic response to calm the person down and lower the heart rate and blood pressure to bring the body back to a state of normal.

If the anxiety is not severe, it can usually be treated naturally by incorporating various relaxation techniques into a daily routine. But severe anxiety should be treated medically and may be done so with a device that sends electrical pulses directly to the vagus nerve.

- **Addiction**

Researchers at the University of Texas, Dallas, School of Behavioral and Brain Sciences, studied breaking the behavioral cycles of addition with vagus nerve stimulation. This research, which began in 2017, found that vagus nerve stimulation supported the 'extinction learning' behavioral pattern of drug-seekers. Stimulating the vagus nerve reduced the cravings better than weaning the user off drugs by slowly reducing their cocaine intake.

Vagus nerve stimulation that was tested on cocaine-addicted lab rats saw a change in the synaptic plasticity connecting the amygdala and the prefrontal cortex. The vagus nerve is stimulated directly by a mild electric current produced by a medical device, approved by the FDA, that gets surgically implanted beneath the skin.

- **Alzheimer's**

The stimulation of the vagus nerve can restore cognitive function. A study that ran from June 2000 to

September 2003 showed that after 1 year of vagus nerve stimulation, most of the 17 patients undergoing the test reported at least no decline from their baseline. While some of the patients showed improvement.

The treatment itself showed that the patients tolerated vagus nerve stimulation well, with no decline or upsets in the patient's quality of life.

- **Autism**

Most patients who have neurodevelopmental disorders have been found to have a low vagal tone. Further studies showed that increasing vagal tone by using Vagus Nerve Stimulation (VNS) can give quite significant improvements in the patient's quality of life after therapy. Along with developmental therapies, VNS could potentially allow the patient to be able to communicate, socialize, and study a lot better.

- **Chronic Fatigue and Fibromyalgia**

Because the vagus nerve regulates many systems in the body, the immune system being one of them, it may be helpful in treating both chronic fatigue syndrome and fibromyalgia.

Vagus nerve stimulation plays a big part in getting rid of pain and is why regular stimulation is useful in helping with the management of fibromyalgia. There are certain areas of the vagus nerve that are responsible for reducing 'temporal summation' which is a process that plays a big part in 'chronic pain states'.

Think of temporal summation as a lasso, parts of the nervous system responsible for pain are lassoed together by temporal summation. Then temporal summation gradually tightens the lasso, and with each squeeze, the body becomes more and more sensitive to pain.

Vagus nerve stimulation has been found to help unwind the central nervous system from the tight embrace of temporal summation to gradually desensitize it to pain.

Chronic fatigue is linked to Fibromyalgia, and the two work in hand and hand. Just as vagus nerve stimulation works to alleviate the symptoms of Fibromyalgia, it can do the same for chronic fatigue syndrome.

- **Depression disorder**

As shown by a study published in 2016, treatment of Major Depressive Disorder (MDD) with vagus nerve stimulation had some positive results. Vagus nerve stimulation improved the connectivity of the Default Mode Network (DMN) in the brain.

- **Epilepsy**

Patients who have received vagus nerve stimulation have reported an improvement in their quality of life. Vagus nerve stimulation decreases the frequency of the seizures as well as the intensity of the seizures. Patients who underwent the therapy have claimed they feel less sleepy during the day and have better cognitive memory.

Vagus nerve therapy for the control of epilepsy is done by a vagus nerve stimulator device. The device is implanted beneath the skin with a wire that runs to the vagus nerve and is wound around it. The device acts similar to that of a pacemaker for the heart, except the VNS stimulator sends mild electrical energy impulses to the brain at regular intervals.

The device operates in such a way that the patient who has the implanted device is not aware of it. If they feel a seizure coming on all they need to do is use a magnet to swipe over the device. This action will send an extra pulse boost which, in turn, may lessen the intensity of the seizure or prevent it altogether.

- **Migraines and Cluster Headaches**

While everyone who suffers from migraines may exhibit some basic similar symptoms, for the most part, no two migraines are alike. They can be anywhere from mild blurred vision, nausea, and discomfort to a full-blown raging pain that makes a person feel like their skull is going to explode. What is worse with this kind of migraine is that if it has developed to this stage there is sure to be nausea and vomiting. Vomiting becomes both a relief and a curse as the pain escalates each time a person vomits.

Vagus nerve therapy was applied in a study as a treatment for chronic migraines and acute cluster headache patients. The non-invasive vagus nerve stimulator targeted the back of the head to stimulate the vagus nerve's cervical branch.

It proved to be effective where most of the patients reported a reduction in pain while others reported no pain at all.

- **OCD and PTSD**

Both OCD and PTSD patients in various trials showed between 40 to 50 % improvement with vagus nerve stimulation. After a year-long trial, patients with OCD, PTSD, and **Personality Disorder (PD)** showed continued improvement with regular treatment and an implanted device.

- **Rheumatoid arthritis**

A study that was conducted in 2016, by experts of immunology in conjunction with neuroscientists on Vagus Nerve Stimulation (VNS), found that the treatment blocked the production of pro-inflammatory cytokines. When pro-inflammatory cytokines cannot be produced it reduces the inflammatory reflex.

This reduces inflammation and cytokines in rheumatoid arthritis patients.

- **Traumatic brain injury**

Traumatic brain injury (TBI) is when some form of injury to the brain causes the neurons to disconnect and then atrophy. Traumatic brain injury has a high mortality rate, especially in military personnel.

There are not many treatments for traumatic brain injury, and depending on the severity, it can leave a person with limited conscious state or in a vegetative state. Upon approval from the FDA to implant vagus nerve stimulators in patients with traumatic brain injury, a study was conducted examining the use of this in TBI patients. This study showed that the stimulation of the vagus nerves affects the stimulation of blood flow to various parts of the brain in order to improve consciousness.

Chapter 5:

HOW TO NATURALLY STIMULATE THE VAGUS NERVE

The only way to directly stimulate the vagus nerve is with a medical device. However, there are natural indirect ways to increase your vagal tone and stimulate the vagus nerve in order to improve physical and mental health.

Acupuncture

Acupuncture is a powerful way to stimulate the vagus nerve. When you choose your acupuncturist, make sure they are a trained and skilled professional. Too much activation of the vagus nerve through acupuncture could also be detrimental to the nerve.

The best place to target is the ears where acupuncture has had a very positive effect on the vagus nerve.

Breathing Exercises

There are certain neurons in the neck and heart that can detect the drop and rise of blood pressure. Taking deep, deliberate breaths from the belly helps to stimulate these receptors, and the receptors will let the Vagus nerve know it needs to regulate the blood pressure. This gets the part of the vagus nerve that deals with the regulation of blood pressure active.

Relax and calmly take around 5-6 deep breaths per minute for around 2 to 3 minutes. Do not overdo it or you could become light-headed and giddy.

Remember to take nice deep breaths in from your belly, hold for a second and release. Do this at least 3 to 4 times a week, if you go to the gym every day, try and concentrate on your breathing while exercising.

You can also use breathing to control pain through the stimulation of your vagus nerve.

Controlling Pain Through Breathing

The Buddhist monks are taught breathing techniques as a way to still the mind and take their focus off things like pain. The mind may seem scattered with thoughts running amok sometimes, but in reality, it can only process one thing at a time.

If we can concentrate on our breath rather than the pain, the body shifts its focus. But the natural human response to pain is to actually hold our breath which automatically switches the body into the sympathetic fight or flight mode.

The same can be said for any kind of pain as stress, anxiety, and fear can come with emotional pain. The type that feels like you have been bruised on the inside and you cannot find the exact center of it or it or how to heal it.

We do not often think about our breathing as it just happens each day naturally. We tend to take it for granted until it shifts and suddenly it is all we can focus on. When this happens, we are usually in a stressful state and the body is in a complete fight or flight mode.

If we can learn to embrace our breath and come to realize just how sacred it is, we can start to learn how to focus our breathing in order to move us away from the pain. Learning to breathe properly has many health benefits including that of increasing vagal tone.

Breathing is a way of quickly calming a person down, and once you know how to focus on your breathing, you can use the technique no matter where you are. But until you have mastered it and are comfortable with it, stick to your quiet peaceful place.

- Sit comfortably, the best position is to sit up straight, legs crossed on a comfortable mat, with your elbows resting comfortably and relaxed on your knees.

- You do not have to close your eyes but to achieve complete focus it is a better option.

- Breath in, taking a deep breath that fills your lungs and extends your belly. Pull your breath into your body for 5 seconds. Try to breathe in through your nose.

- Hold for 1 to 2 seconds then slowly let the breath move back out of your body.

- Count to 5 and repeat the breathing as you do concentrate on the breath going into your body. Filling each cell with oxygen as the mind, body, and soul start to relax.

- As you breathe out, try to think about the breath leaving your body carrying all the stress, anxiety, worry, and pain out of your system.

- Try to get to around 7 breaths per minute (the average intake is 14 breaths per minute). This ensures that your nervous system has switched to parasympathetic mode as it starts to relax the mind and body.

- More oxygen supply to the body and brain also means that the body starts to feel good, when the body starts to feel good it releases all the feel-good hormones like endorphins.

- Conscious breathing exercises have been around for centuries and can help to lower blood pressure, stress, anxiety, and pain levels. All without the nasty side effects that conventional medication would have.

Chanting

In 2011, the International Journal of Yoga conducted a study on 'OM' chanting. The study compared chanting the classic 'OM' with 'SSS' to determine which chant would be more effective in stimulating the vagus nerve.

The chanting of 'OM' has a vibration effect on the ears as well as the vocal cords, which is in turn sent to the vagus nerve. This information reaches the vagus nerve through the auricular and deactivates the limbic system to produce peace and calm within the body.

How to Chant

- Go to a quiet space, one where there is no disturbing noise and there is only peace.

- Some people like the gentle sound of trickling water or a soft chirp of a bird. Find your quiet space.

- The floor is the best space to sit as it brings you closer to the earth and centers you.

- Make sure you are comfortable; the best position is to sit with your legs folded in front of you like you are going to meditate. If you cannot find a position that works for you or if you cannot sit on the floor, sit in a chair with your legs in a comfortable position.

- Your elbows need to be able to be positioned in a relaxed state in order to hold your mudra (hand positioning).

- There are a few ways to position your hands while chanting. The positioning of your hands is what determines how you hold your mind and the flow of energy throughout your body.

- The most common position for the hands is to hold your thumb and index fingers on each hand in an O, sit with your palms turned up. This is called the Jnana Mudra and is known as the wisdom seal. It is used to create a feeling of energy, light, and upliftment.

- When you are settled, start to relax your mind, body, and soul by concentrating on your breathing.

- Close your eyes and take slow steady breaths by breathing in through your nose and out through your mouth.

- When you are ready to start chanting, take a steady breath in. Then as you release your breath out, start to chant the 'OM' by holding the 'O' for 5 seconds then the 'M' for another 5 seconds.

- As you release your breath and chant, let the sense of wisdom start to manifest and grow within the palms of your hands.

- Chant for 10 to 15 minutes in order to achieve a clear state of mind and a good workout for your vagus nerve.

- End your chant with grace and gratitude, remembering to breathe.

Cold

Exposure to the cold stimulates both your sympathetic and parasympathetic systems. When you first step into the cold, your body's first response is to flee back into the warmth. But as your systems adapt to the cold, your body's fight and flight response is calmed down and counteracted by the 'rest-and-digest' response from the parasympathetic system which is overseen by the vagus nerve.

You don't have to get hypothermia for the nerve to be stimulated, you just need to be out in the cold long enough to do the trick. You can do this by:

- Dipping your full face into cold water for a few seconds at a time. Make sure your entire face from below the chin to the top of the hairline on your forehead is submerged in the water. Do this 3 or 4 times holding each dunk for 2 to 4 seconds. This form of cold submergence is effective for switching the body into parasympathetic mode after strenuous exercise, a bad upset, a scare, or when you are over-anxious, angry, or feeling tired.

- Taking a cold shower for around 30 seconds to a minute, you must let the cold spray cover your entire body from head to toe.

- Stand outside in the fresh snow for 30 seconds to 2 minutes (do snow angels or build a snowman for longer exposure).

- Drinking a nice cold glass of water or sucking on an ice cube can also work.

Coughing

When coughing hard, it will generate pressure in your chest and this, in turn, stimulate the vagus nerve. Be careful not to do it too many times though as you do not want to hurt your throat or damage it.

Exercising

Mild exercise can also help stimulate the vagus nerve as it stimulates a lot of organs and muscles, and affects breathing, heart rate, and blood pressure, all of which have some effect on the vagus nerve.

When exercising, keep your fitness level in mind and work to what you are comfortable with, gradually increasing at a steady pace. Going all out, all at once, does more damage than good.

Try the following exercises or practices:

- A brisk walk 4 to 5 times a week for at least 20 to 30 minutes. Wear comfortable shoes and clothes, remember to concentrate on your breathing and posture. While you are walking, rather than put yourself in harm's way by blocking out what is going on around you, ditch the music and headset. Take note of your surroundings, hum, or sing as you go. Look for new things each day on your walk, take in all the beauty that is around you. Literally, stop to smell the roses.

- Aqua-aerobics 2 to 3 times a week. Water stimulates a lot of senses in your body, it is also where your body feels at ease as you were grown in a fluid. It also allows you to take deep breaths and concentrate on your breathing.

- Swimming for a few minutes each day even in the winter (for cold stimulation) is a good way to get your nerve centers active, increase your fitness, and enhance your feeling of well-being.

- Weightlifting is also a good way to stimulate the vagus nerve. Be careful not to overdo it, try to get the advice of a qualified trainer and build up your muscle strength as you build your vagus nerve tone.

- Stretching out and flexing your muscles, taking nice deep breaths and pulling in the abdomen.

- Yoga is another great way to center yourself and get the balance back into your life. It strengthens, it tones, it leans, and it helps you breathe correctly.

- A sport such as baseball, softball, soccer, hockey, netball, basketball, and ice skating. These all get the adrenaline flowing, they put the body into an excited state without feeling too threatened.

- Tai Chi works to center the body and teaches you to be aware of each part of yourself. The smooth easy relaxed flow while exercising the body and mind is a great way to stimulate the vagus nerve.

- Dance is a way to get your body's energy flowing, it is a great way to relieve stress and music really does soothe the soul.

Eating Correctly and Adding Supplements

There are some foods that are more helpful for stimulating the vagus nerve than others.

- Eat more fish in your diet. Fish has nutrients in it that help to lower the heart rate as well as increase the heart rate variability. If you are not a big fan of fish, then try natural fish oil supplements instead.

- There are receptors in the brain called GABA receptors, they are responsible for mood changes. Taking probiotics on a regular basis helps with these GABA receptors and has a positive effect on a person's mood.

- Zinc, try and get a bit more zinc in your system as it helps with vagal toning.

- Eat fiber on a regular basis as fiber has a positive effect on the gut, it also helps to keep a person feeling fuller for longer.

- Chew gum, while it may be considered a bad habit and frowned upon by some, chewing gum actually gets the brain to release a hormone called cholecystokinin or CCK. CCK is a hormone that the body releases once you have eaten in order to aid digestion. When you chew gum, the body is getting ready to digest whatever you have in your mouth. Be careful when you choose your gum, make sure it is good for your teeth and not too high in sugar, that it doesn't contain harmful colorants, etc. Also, never swallow gum as your body cannot digest it correctly.

Fasting

Fasting is good for both the metabolism and the vagus nerve. When you fast, it slows down the metabolism. This is done by the Vagus nerve. Be sure to check with a medical professional before you make any changes to your diet if you have a preexisting condition. People who suffer from low blood pressure must take extra care. Fasting can significantly lower blood pressure, which is dangerous for those whose blood pressure is already low.

Fasting should be set out by a registered dietician or a medical professional in order to incorporate it correctly into your lifestyle.

Gag Reflex

One way a doctor checks for damage to the vagus nerve is to test your gag reflex. You can also stimulate your vagus nerve by prompting your gag reflex. Do not do it too many times in one sitting as you may encourage vomiting and could damage your gag reflex. Try not to do it too often either, maybe go for 2 to 3 times a month.

You can use a cotton bud, a tongue depressor, your toothbrush, or your finger. Be careful when using your finger or anything hard at the back of your throat as it is easy to nick and damage the soft tissue which can cause an infection.

Gargle

Try to gargle something such as mouthwash, saltwater, or even normal water will do. Gargling gets the muscles in the back of the throat working by contracting these muscles. As soon as they contract, they trigger the vagus nerve which in turn will stimulate the GI tract.

Humming

Humming causes gentle vibrations along the Vagus nerve which stimulate it. It is also something that gives people a feel-good happy vibe which is also good stimulation for Vagus nerve stimulation. It also exercises parts of the vocal cords and throat.

Knees to Chest

Sit on a mat or your bed, take a deep breath and then lift your knees up to your chest and hold them there for 1 minute. Take another deep breath and extend your legs then stretch out your body.

Repeat this for 3 to 4 times. It is an exercise you can do each morning when you wake up and before you go to bed. It makes your whole body feel relaxed and warm, plus it stimulates the vagus nerve.

Laugh More

Laughter has many, many health benefits. Even smiling on its own is beneficial to your health and there is nothing catchier than a smile. Nine out of ten times when you see someone laughing merrily you will get a smile on your face or you will join in on the merriment.

Smiling and laughing have been proven to lower your heart rate and blood pressure, it also makes you look more attractive, appealing, and reliable to others. Another way to stimulate your vagus nerve is to build better relationships with others, smiling at another person is a way of creating a symbiotic connection. As you smile at a person their brain has an automatic response that usually coaxes them to smile back at you.

There are times when you just do not feel like smiling and it will feel like the hardest thing to do but try it anyway. Lift up the edges of your mouth and do it, even if no one is watching. Better yet, smile at yourself in the mirror. Make your brain create that connection and you will feel a lot better.

Smiling and laughter is not a magic cure for everything, but it is one of the best medicines for stress relief. It also stimulates your vagus nerve as it increases the heart rate variation. It can also be one of the side effects that some people may have by stimulating the vagus nerve.

There is a syndrome that is quite rare called Angelman's syndrome, this syndrome causes people to pass out when they are tickled. Angelman's syndrome has been associated with the stimulation of the vagus nerve.

Massage

There are many types of massage you can have or do to stimulate the vagus nerve. A massage can stimulate the vagus nerve which is good for heart health as well as your digestive health.

- A foot massage is one of the best massages, as your feet are an important part of your anatomy. If you are not feeling well or if you are not looking after them properly, it can negatively affect many aspects of your health and wellbeing. A good foot massage can stimulate the vagus nerve regulating your heart rate and blood pressure.

- A deep tissue massage from a trained professional will stimulate many nerves in the body, including the vagus nerve which can increase circulation, oxygenation, and relaxation.

- A carotid sinus massage can stimulate the vagus nerve, however, this massage should only ever be done by a trained medical professional. It is usually done to control seizures.

- Massage the back of the neck, this releases stress and tension in the muscles of the neck.

- Massage the ear lobes as this can have a nice soothing and relaxing effect on the body.

Meditation

It is a good way to increase a person's energy, slow down the heart rate, blood pressure, relieve stress, relieve pain, lower anxiety, regulate your breathing, and increase blood circulation.

In a meditative state, the vagus nerve signals that the body is in a safe state. This is a great way to get the body out a stuck state of fight or flight and back into homeostasis.

Natural Vitamin D (Sunlight)

Sitting in the sun for limited periods of time (with a good sunblock, a hat, and sunglasses) boosts the activation of certain hormones that are good for stimulating the vagus nerve.

Sunlight is good for a lot of other things as well, it gives you a feeling of well-being and can literally brighten your entire day. The sun is kind of like the sky smiling down on you, you feel all warm inside and out.

This feeling of well-being in itself is a great source of stimulation for the vagus nerve.

Salivate

If you are able to create a lot of saliva in your mouth it means that you have successfully activated your vagus nerve. In order for the body to produce a lot of saliva, it has to be in the parasympathetic mode which means that the body needs to be in a calm relaxed state to fill the mouth with saliva.

If you are struggling to do this go relax in a place where you feel calm, close your eyes and think of squeezing a lime or lemon into your mouth.

Breathe deeply and relax the tongue in the warm saliva, the more relaxed you become the more saliva your mouth will be able to produce. You should feel a state of calm in about 3 to 5 minutes.

Sing

Singing is a quick way to vibrate and stimulate the vocal cords which are managed by the vagus nerve

Singing does a lot of good for a person and has quite a few positive effects on the vagus nerve. It exercises the back of the throat, it keeps a person in a calm state, and when people sing in unison it makes them feel more connected to each other.

Singing increases a hormone called oxytocin which is better known as the love hormone, this stimulates all the other feel-good hormones and is like a complete boost of activity for the vagus nerve.

So, sing and dance like no one is watching as it is good for your health and vagal tone.

Sleeping and Sleeping Properly

Sleep! Lack of sleep and sleep disorders can negatively affect the vagus nerve. So, you need to get in some good quality sleep.

To get good quality sleep you may have to train your body to go to sleep and wake up at consistent times. Or at least set a sleep window where you have at least six good hours of sleep a night. But 7 to 9 hours is a lot better, although not always achievable for parents, people with hectic jobs, and people with sleep disorders.

But there are a few things you can do to optimize your sleep environment to help you achieve a decent quality of sleep.

- Make sure your room is dark, there should be no light that is shining directly on you. Light on any kind makes your brain think it is still daytime, that is why in a baby's room you should have blackout blinds for their daytime naps, it helps them fall asleep faster and sleep deeper.

- Make sure there are no devices like laptops or smartphones in the room. They constantly emit a blue light, which is the worst kind of light to have in your bedroom. If you need your phone, there are various apps you can download that can stop the phone from emitting this light.

- Don't have a TV in the room. You may think it helps you fall asleep but subconsciously, your brain is still aware of what is happening on the television.

- Rather, read before going to bed instead of watching TV, and by reading, we mean an actual book. A book that has real paper pages.

- Make sure you have the right pillow that supports your head and neck to align your spine comfortably.

- Make sure your mattress is comfortable for you. If you wake up with bad pins and needles or feeling numb, it is time to change your mattress.

- Set the temperature in your room to be cool but not too cold. The best temperature is around 20°C or 70°F. If it is too hot you struggle to sleep, too cold and you struggle to sleep, it has to be just right.

- Try and eliminate as much noise as possible to make your bedroom quiet and peaceful. Remember, even when you are sleeping your subconscious is aware of all the noise around you.

- Sleep on your right side — sleeping on your right increases your variable heart rates, keeps your blood pressure low, and offers the most vagus nerve activity. Try to avoid sleeping on your back or stomach as these have the lowest vagus nerve activations.

- If you exercise during the day, it relieves stress and ensures a good night's sleep.

- Make a conscious effort to leave problems, worries, and troubles at the bedroom door.

- Watch what you eat before you go to bed and avoid stimulants before sleeping, like coffee.

- Keep a glass of water next to your bed but try not to consume too much water during the night or before bed or you will have to get up during the night.

- Use your meditation techniques to relax your mind, body, and soul to drift off.

Relaxation

Probably one of the best ways to keep your vagus nerve healthy is knowing how to relax and unwind.

Here are some exercises to help you relax:

- The body scan

  - Lie back on your bed or recline in your favorite comfy chair as long as you can extend your body.

  - Make sure your arms are at your sides, your legs are straight out and extended with your head cushioned comfortably.

  - Close your eyes and center yourself by taking a few deep cleansing breaths.

  - Take a deep breath in and feel it moving all the way down from your head down to your toes.

  - As you slowly let it out, stretch your toes out and then your feet as you picture your breath leaving each muscle like your calves, then your knees, then your torso. As it does, tense them and release them all the way through your fingers and then out your mouth.

○ It is important to gently tense each body part as you make your way up, hold it for a second then release it.

○ The scan goes:

- toes

- Feet and ankles

- Calves

- Knees

- Thighs

- Buttocks

- Lower stomach

- Upper stomach

- Chest

- Fingers

- Hands

- Forearms

- Upper arms

- Neck

- Flex the ears

- Breath out the mouth

  ○ Repeat the process 3 to 5 times

- Open your imagination

Another trick is to take your mind on a magical journey where there is only peace, calm, and things that fill your imagination with happiness.

- Chamomile, a good book, a cozy chair, and a quiet corner

There is nothing better than curling up with a good book and a cup of chamomile tea to relax a person. Not only does it relax you it also stimulates your brain, keeping it healthy like doing Sudoku or crossword puzzles, it exercises the memory muscle.

Socialize

Socializing helps your body function on a social level without feeling threatened at every turn. In order for the body to be able to maintain homeostasis, you have to be able to work at all levels. This includes socializing, which is a big part of life. You cannot go to the shops without some form of socializing.

A good healthy relationship with friends, family, and loved ones keeps the body at ease as no matter where you are, you feel as if you have a safety net. This enables you to go out and form other connections in the world.

Positive relationships start at home even if that home is with your best friend.

Conclusion

It is a horrible feeling when you feel you are trapped by the body's inability to work as it should or as a prisoner of your mind. But we do have the power to take back the control, after all, we are the true command center, and we can start to do that by getting our vagus nerve back into shape.

As with any transformation, this process comes with some sort of change. If you are willing to make a few lifestyle adjustments and work on your vagus nerve, you will soon start to feel better and reap the benefits.

It is best to remember that nothing is going to magically happen overnight, and it will take a few days or weeks to start to feel the changes. The trick is not to give up and to persevere, and you should feel the rewards of your hard work.

If you have a pre-existing medical condition, always check with your doctor or health care advisor before you implement the changes. You don't have to have any preexisting medical conditions to want to get in shape or to ensure your body is at its peak in order to be able to take on stressful situations with ease.

Implementing a few lifestyle changes is healthy for anyone and exercising or stimulating your vagus nerve is a great way to ensure your body's resilience and health.

Made in the USA
Middletown, DE
07 September 2020

19028527R10071